IØ117192

The Quiet Unravelling

Understanding and Recovering from Burnout and Compassion Fatigue

Author: Andrea Pluck   Cover page by Jeremy Pluck

Cover image: Unravelling 2 Sculpture, hand formed aluminium wire, 2024

Artist: Louise Daniels (www.danielsvisualarts.com)

Photograph: Dylan Proctor

First published in 2025 in Australia by Publisher:
Pluck Pluck Goose
1 Vaucluse Crescent, Bellevue Heights 5050,   P P G
South Australia

ISBN: 978-0-9756253-7-8

9 780975 625378

Introduction

Burnout rarely kicks down the door.

It slips in softly, almost unnoticed. A yawn that stretches too long. A session that takes a little more out of you than usual. A reluctance to return a call, open an email, or show up fully in a space you once loved. Slowly—almost imperceptibly—you begin to feel distant from yourself, like you are showing up in your own life in faded tones. The work you once felt passionate about becomes something you *push through*. The care you once offered freely now feels like a weight.

This is the quiet unravelling. And if you are reading this, you might already know it all too well.

You might be a therapist, health professional, carer, educator—or simply someone who cares deeply. People who offer themselves in service of others are especially vulnerable to burnout and compassion fatigue, not because we are weak, but because we are wired to care. It is our superpower... and sometimes, our undoing.

It is not a checklist or a lecture. It is a companion to walk beside you as you start to recognise what is happening, reflect on how you got here, and gently explore the path forward.

Together, we will look at:

What burnout and compassion fatigue really are (and what they are not).

How to spot the early signs before they become a full-blown collapse.

Why traditional self-care advice often falls short.

What recovery can look like (no, it is not just bubble baths and saying no more often).

How to reconnect with meaning, purpose, and energy—without abandoning your compassionate nature.

In this book there will be stories. Reflections. Gentle prompts. And above all, permission to feel what you feel, to rest, to reclaim your inner life, and to find your way back to yourself.

Whether you are reading this from the bottom of the burnout well or just sensing that something's off, I hope this book feels like a deep exhale. You are not broken. You are not failing. You are just human.

And it is time to come home.

About the Author

Andrea Pluck is a passionate massage therapist, educator, and writer dedicated to supporting therapists, healers, and caregivers in their personal and professional wellbeing journeys. Drawing from her extensive experience in remedial massage and lymphatic care, Andrea blends evidence-based practice with compassionate storytelling to create resources that uplift and empower.

She believes that caring for those who care for others is essential to building sustainable healing communities. Andrea's work shines a light on burnout and compassion fatigue, offering practical tools and heartfelt wisdom to help others reclaim their strength, boundaries, and joy.

When she's not writing or teaching, Andrea enjoys exploring nature, practicing mindfulness, and sipping good coffee while dreaming up new ways to make wellbeing accessible to all.

A Personal Note from the Author

I didn't realise I was burned out at first. Like many therapists and caregivers, I thought I was just tired, maybe a bit overworked. I told myself it would pass—that I just needed a weekend, a good sleep, a little holiday. But the truth was getting louder each day.

One morning, I found myself sitting in my car in the work car park, hands on the wheel, keys in the ignition—but unable to move. My body was frozen, but my mind was racing. I was trying to psych myself up just to walk into the building. Not for anything dramatic—just to start a normal day. And I couldn't do it. I felt numb and wired at the same time. The thought of smiling, caring, or answering one more email felt like trying to lift a mountain.

That moment didn't come out of nowhere. It was the result of months—years—of giving more than I had to give, of pushing through warning signs, of believing that rest was a luxury and that boundaries were for people who weren't "committed enough."

That moment, sitting in my car, was the quiet unravelling. Not dramatic. Not obvious to anyone else. But it was my signal that something had to change.

I wrote it for you—because I know what it is like to lose your spark and feel like you are still obligated to push through. I know the guilt, the exhaustion, the fear of not being enough.

If you are reading this and nodding, this book is for you.

"Sometimes the most courageous thing we can do is to stop."

— Brené Brown

Contents

Chapter 1: Not Lazy. Not Broken.

Redefining Burnout and Compassion Fatigue

We don't wake up one day and think, "Ah yes, today is the day I burn out."

It looks like sighing at emails. Forgetting simple things. Feeling numb where you used to feel joy. You are tired, but sleep doesn't fix it. You want rest but can't seem to take it. And somewhere along the way, a little voice whispers, "Maybe you are just not cut out for this after all."

Let me stop you right there.

You are not lazy. You are not weak.

And you are most definitely not broken. You are tired in a way that runs deep—in your bones, in your spirit, in the parts of you that care the most. That kind of tired doesn't get better with a nap. It needs recognition, gentleness, and space to breathe.

Let's start by understanding what this really is.

The Slow Unravel, Not the Sudden Crash

Burnout doesn't usually hit all at once. It's more like an unravelling — slow and silent — as the threads that once held you together begin to come undone.

You don't just stop showing up. You keep going. You keep doing. You smile. You answer calls. You show up to your job, your family, your responsibilities. But underneath, something's changing. You are detached. Going through the motions. Your body is present, but your mind and heart feel far away.

Burnout and compassion fatigue don't mean you are doing something wrong. They mean something has gone out of balance—often for too long.

It is a mismatch between effort and replenishment. Between the energy you give and the support you receive. Between the care you offer and the care you allow yourself to take (Figley, 2002).

Burnout vs. Compassion Fatigue vs. Depression

These terms are often tossed around interchangeably, but they are distinct—even if they overlap.

Burnout is a state of emotional, physical, and mental exhaustion caused by prolonged stress, usually related to work or caregiving. The World Health Organization (2019) classifies burnout as an occupational phenomenon—not a medical condition—but acknowledges its profound impact. It is defined by three dimensions:

- Exhaustion
- Mental distance or negativity related to one's job
- Reduced professional efficacy

Compassion fatigue, often described as "the cost of caring," occurs when continuous exposure to others' suffering leads to emotional depletion. It can result in emotional numbing, irritability, and a decreased ability to empathise (Figley, 2002; Huggard et al., 2022). It is common among therapists, nurses, carers, teachers, and even parents—anyone in a sustained helping role.

Depression is a diagnosable mental illness characterised by persistent low mood, anhedonia (loss of interest in previously enjoyable activities), and cognitive and physical symptoms that impair functioning across multiple areas of life (American Psychiatric Association [APA], 2022).

Intersections and Implications

Understanding the distinctions between burnout, compassion fatigue, and depression is crucial for accurate diagnosis and effective intervention. While they share some overlapping symptoms, their causes, manifestations, and treatment approaches differ. Recognizing these differences can aid in developing targeted strategies for prevention and recovery.

Burnout and compassion fatigue can coexist with, or lead to, depression—but they are not the same thing. (*Burnout, compassion fatigue, depression—what's the difference?* DVM360).

If you are unsure which applies to you, or you suspect you may be experiencing depression, please speak with a qualified mental health professional. You don't need to figure this out alone.

Common Myths That Keep Us Stuck

Let's name a few persistent myths that sneak into our tired brains:

Myth 1: "If I were stronger, I'd be fine."

Truth: Burnout is not a failure of character. It is often the result of unrelenting demands combined with inadequate support (Maslach & Leiter, 2016). It affects the most dedicated, conscientious individuals—especially those who care deeply.

Myth 2: "Other people have it worse, I should be grateful."

Truth: Gratitude does not negate struggle. Minimising your pain because someone else is suffering more only adds shame to exhaustion. Compassion fatigue thrives in comparison and silence (Sinclair et al., 2017).

Myth 3: "I just need a better routine/mindset/time management system."

Truth: Burnout recovery is not about colour-coded calendars. While habits help, real healing often requires structural change: boundaries, rest, delegation, and sometimes stepping away entirely (West et al., 2018).

Myth 4: "Self-care will fix it."

Truth: Self-care is essential, but insufficient on its own. Recovery from burnout needs community, boundaries, and systemic change—not just massages and magnesium (Hersey, 2022).

You are Not the Problem

Burnout is not a personal failure. It is a natural response to chronic overload and emotional labour. When the system is broken, the people in it break, too.

You are not the problem. The fact that you feel so deeply and care so much is a gift. It just needs tending. Boundaries. Space. And support.

Let this be a reminder. You are not broken. You are tired. And there is a way forward.

Reflection

To deepen your understanding and begin the journey toward healing, consider the following:

Recognising the Signs

What signs have shown up in your body, mind, or relationships that something might be off?

Exploring Personal Myths

Which beliefs about strength or productivity have kept you pushing past your limits?

Assessing Support

Where do you receive support—and where do you feel unsupported?

Identifying Needs

What does your nervous system need more of? What does it need less of?

Setting Gentle Intentions

What is one thing you can do this week to acknowledge your exhaustion without trying to fix it?

Chapter 2: The Science of Exhaustion

How Burnout Affects the Brain, Body, and Nervous System

Burnout is not just "in your head." It is in your hormones. It is in your immune system. It is in your memory lapses, your gut issues, your aching joints, and your rattled nerves.

When you live in a prolonged state of physical and emotional overload, your body adapts—at first helpfully, then harmfully. The science of burnout is really the science of **stress without relief**.

Let's take a closer look at the biology and explore how chronic stress rewires your brain, hijacks your nervous system, and slowly chips away at your capacity to feel, think, sleep, and even care.

Your Stress System, Explained Simply

Your body is designed to handle stress—briefly.

When you encounter a threat—real or perceived—your **sympathetic nervous system** kicks into gear. Adrenaline floods your system. Your heart races. Muscles tense. Digestion halts. Blood vessels constrict, causing your blood pressure to rise. You are primed to run, fight, or freeze.

Once the threat is over, your **parasympathetic nervous system** is meant to bring things back to baseline: slowing your heart, deepening your breath, calming your mind.

Burnout begins when that "recovery phase" never arrives.

Your body stays stuck in **go-mode** for too long. Cortisol (the stress hormone) remains elevated. Over time, your ability to self-regulate diminishes—and your nervous system becomes like a fire alarm that won't turn off.

Key Study: Research by McEwen (2004) introduced the concept of **allostatic load**—the cumulative wear and tear on the body from chronic stress. High allostatic load has been linked to memory issues, fatigue, poor immunity, and even heart disease.

Brain on Burnout: What Changes

Burnout doesn't just make you feel foggy—it *literally* affects your brain.

The Prefrontal Cortex (your rational, decision-making centre) shows reduced activity during burnout. That's why tasks feel harder, memory gets patchy, and decision fatigue sets in (Golkar et al., 2014).

The Amygdala (your brain's alarm centre) becomes more reactive. You are more likely to over-respond to stress and misread safe situations as threatening.

The Hippocampus (involved in learning and memory) shrinks in size with prolonged stress—affecting emotional regulation and recall (Savic, 2015).

Burnout doesn't make you broken—it rewires your brain for survival. But brains are plastic. With rest and support, this wiring can change again.

The brain's neuroplasticity allows it to adapt. With rest and support the brain can adapt positively. (Bay Area CBT Center. (2025). *Neuroplasticity: Harnessing your brain's ability to adapt and thrive.*)

The Role of the Vagus Nerve: Your Built-In Recovery Tool

The **vagus nerve** is like your body's brake pedal. It helps regulate digestion, heart rate, mood, and immune function. When you hum, sigh, laugh, or breathe deeply, you are activating your **parasympathetic system** via the vagus nerve.

Low **vagal tone** (a sign of underactive parasympathetic response) has been found in people experiencing burnout, depression, and trauma (Porges, 2011).

Practices that gently stimulate the vagus nerve—like slow breathing, singing, cold exposure, and connection—can support recovery from chronic stress (Streeter et al., 2012).

Immune System & Inflammation

When stress becomes chronic, your immune system goes from "vigilant" to "vulnerable."

Elevated cortisol initially suppresses inflammation. But over time, the body may become **cortisol-resistant**—leading to **chronic low-grade**

inflammation that's associated with fatigue, pain, and even autoimmune flare-ups (Juster et al., 2010).

You may find yourself catching every cold, healing slowly, or dealing with flare-ups of pre-existing health conditions. This is not "all in your head"—it is happening on a cellular level.

Sleep, Digestion & Hormones

Burnout can sabotage the body's core repair systems:

Sleep: High cortisol disrupts melatonin production, making it harder to fall or stay asleep—even when you are exhausted (Meerlo et al., 2008).

Digestion: Chronic stress inhibits digestion, alters gut bacteria, and can lead to bloating, reflux, and IBS-like symptoms (Konturek et al., 2011).

Hormones: Stress affects everything from sex hormones to blood sugar regulation. People experiencing burnout may notice irregular periods, libido changes, weight fluctuations, or worsened PMS.

Reflection

Take a moment to explore how burnout may be showing up in your own body:

Body Awareness

What physical symptoms have you been experiencing that may be connected to stress?

Sleep and Rest

Are you able to fall asleep easily? Do you stay asleep? Do you wake feeling rested?

Nervous System Check-In

When was the last time you truly felt safe, relaxed, and unhurried?

Are there small practices that help you shift from "on alert" to "at ease"?

Can you observe your symptoms with curiosity instead of judgment?

What is one new way you might support your body's recovery this week?

Chapter 3: The Hidden Cost of Caring

The Emotional Toll of Caregiving and Why It Often Goes Unseen

Caregiving is considered a noble act — the heart of so many professions and relationships. But beneath the surface, the relentless giving takes a toll that is rarely acknowledged or understood.

Whether you are a therapist, nurse, massage therapist, parent, or friend, caring for others can quietly drain your emotional reserves.

This chapter shines a light on the invisible price caregivers pay, including emotional labour, blurred boundaries, and the pervasive myth that self-sacrifice is the only way.

Caregivers are the ones who answer the midnight calls.
Who hold the space.
Who carry the worries.
Who show up, again and again, heart-first.

But who shows up for them?

Whether you are a therapist, a nurse, a massage practitioner, a teacher, a parent, a volunteer, or simply *the one everyone leans on*, caregiving becomes more than a task. It becomes an identity. A quiet contract: *I will hold this for you. Even when I'm tired. Even when no one sees.*

When carers become emotionally, physically, and spiritually depleted, the impact can be profound—yet often overlooked. There is a hidden toll of emotional labour, the unspoken cost of always being the strong one, and the damaging belief that caring for others must come at the expense of caring for ourselves.

Emotional Labour: The Work Behind the Work

The term **emotional labour**, coined by sociologist Arlie Hochschild (1983), describes the effort involved in managing emotions to meet the expectations of a role—often in service professions.

Massage therapists are expected to be calm and compassionate. Nurses must remain composed in the face of trauma. Teachers absorb the emotions of their students while maintaining order. Parents juggle patience with exhaustion.

This invisible work—so often gendered, so often unacknowledged—is exhausting. Over time, it can lead to what researchers now call **emotional exhaustion**, a core component of burnout (Maslach & Leiter, 2016).

And get this: you don't have to be officially employed to experience emotional labour. If you've ever smiled through your own pain to keep someone else afloat, you've done it.

The Helper Identity Trap

Many caregivers don't just *do* caring work—they *are* caregivers. Their sense of worth, safety, or identity may be deeply entwined with helping.

On the surface, it looks noble. But underneath, it can become a trap.

"If I stop helping, who am I?"

"If I say no, will they still need me?"

"If I rest, am I selfish?"

This mindset can create a dangerous loop: the more depleted you become, the more you push yourself to prove your value. You override your own needs to maintain the role—and in doing so, abandon the very care you offer others.

Researchers call this the **compassion fatigue cycle**: a pattern of overextending, numbing, and continuing to give without receiving support (Figley, 2002; Huggard et al., 2022).

Boundary Erosion and Empathic Distress

Caregivers often have blurred boundaries—not from lack of skill, but from **chronic over-exposure to other people's needs**.

In trauma-impacted professions (or families), it becomes normal to:

- Cancel your own plans to help others
- Ignore early signs of your own exhaustion
- Take responsibility for others' emotions

Over time, this leads to **empathic distress**—when your ability to care becomes a source of pain (Singer & Klimecki, 2014). You begin to shut down, not because you don't care, but because your nervous system is overwhelmed.

"Why am I irritated all the time?"

"Why does even a simple request feel like too much?"

"Why can't I seem to feel anything at all?"

These are not failures of empathy. They're survival mechanisms. They're signals that you need tending, too.

They don't call care-giving self-sacrificing for nothing. You really are sacrificing yourself.

The Myth of Martyrdom

We're often taught to value selflessness above all else—even at our own expense.

To be the one who keeps going.
The one who never says no.
The one who sacrifices everything for others.

But the martyr model of care is unsustainable. It teaches us that burnout is noble, and that boundaries are selfish.

The truth? **Sustainable care requires reciprocity.** You are not a machine. You are not a bottomless well. You are a living system—one that needs rest, play, affection, and care to function.

And you deserve those things **not because you have earned them through service**—but because you are human.

Reflection

Take a moment to turn your attention inward:

What do you believe about saying no?

When is it hardest for you to set boundaries? What fears come up?

How do you know when you are overextended?

What are your early warning signs—physical, emotional, or behavioural?

Where do you receive care, if at all?

Is there someone or something that helps you refill your emotional cup?

What do you fear might happen if you stopped always being the strong one?

Can you imagine a version of support that includes you, too?

Chapter 4: Spotting the Cracks

Early Signs, Red Flags, and When to Take Action

If you're reading this, chances are you're someone who gives generously—to your clients, your community, your loved ones. And perhaps, over time, that giving has quietly overshadowed your own needs. Not out of neglect, but out of habit. Out of heart. But even the most giving soul needs to be held. Even you. Especially you.

This chapter is about tuning into those small shifts in your feelings, your energy, your behaviour—that say you might be running low. Spotting these cracks early is not about being perfect or fixing everything at once. It is about being gentle with yourself and honouring what you need.

Why Paying Attention Matters

Think of it this way: If your phone battery starts to flicker low, you plug it in. If your car makes a strange noise, you get it checked. Your mind and body deserve the same attention and care. Those small signals—

your "flat battery lights"—are invitations to pause and listen.

Catching these signs early gives you space to breathe, to take small, manageable steps before things feel too heavy.

Physical Signals: Your Body Speaks First

Your body is wise. It notices stress before your mind even registers it. Maybe you are feeling tired in a way that sleep doesn't fix, or you notice tension creeping into your neck and shoulders like an unwelcome guest. Perhaps your sleep has become restless, or your stomach churns more often than usual.

This is your body asking for kindness. When fatigue becomes your constant companion, or headaches settle in like old friends who overstay their welcome, it is time to pause and check in with yourself.

Emotional and Mental Signals

Emotionally, you might feel like you are on a rollercoaster without the fun. Maybe little things frustrate you more than they should, or you find yourself feeling numb where once there was joy.

It is okay to admit that your heart feels heavy, or that your motivation has dimmed. These feelings are not signs of weakness or failure—they're the natural response of a heart that's been giving too much without enough refilling.

Sometimes, you might feel distant from your work or the people you care for, like you are watching life from behind a glass wall. That's compassion fatigue quietly building its weight.

Changes in Behaviour: What You Might Not Notice

You might start to pull back—skipping social outings, avoiding friends, or saying "no" more often (and sometimes feeling guilty about it). Maybe your usual routines, like exercise or mealtimes, begin to slip. Or perhaps you lean into habits that offer quick comfort but leave you feeling emptier later—extra coffee, late-night scrolling, or a glass (or two) of wine.

These behaviours are not flaws or failures—they're signs you are trying to cope the best way you know how.

Cognitive Fog and Decision Fatigue

Burnout can cloud your thinking. Tasks that once felt simple might now seem overwhelming. You might find your mind wandering, forgetting appointments, or struggling to make even small decisions.

This fog is not a reflection of your intelligence or worth—it is your brain signalling that it is tired and needs rest.

Recognising Compassion Fatigue

If you are someone who gives emotionally, you might feel a creeping numbness towards the people you care for. You might dread going to work or feel overwhelmed just thinking about your next session or caregiving task.

These feelings are heartbreaking but more common than you might think—and they don't mean you don't care. They mean your heart needs healing and space to breathe.

Gentle Check-In

Take a quiet moment with these questions. There are no right or wrong answers—just what is true for you right now.

1. What is your body telling you? Are there aches, pains, or exhaustion that you've been pushing aside?

2. How have your emotions shifted lately? Are there feelings you've been avoiding or minimizing?

3. Have you noticed changes in how you interact with others or take care of yourself?

4. What thoughts keep circling in your mind? Are they kind or critical?

5. When do you feel most drained? When do you feel even a flicker of energy or joy?

6. Who or what helps you feel safe and supported?

You deserve to listen to your own answers with kindness.

When to Reach Out

If these cracks have started to feel like gaps, it is time to reach out. This might mean talking to a trusted friend, a professional, or taking a break from your usual responsibilities. Asking for help is one of the bravest and kindest things you can do—not just for yourself, but for everyone who depends on you.

You don't have to do this alone.

A Story of Early Recognition

Anna, a massage therapist I've known for years, was always known for her warmth and empathy. Over months, she noticed subtle changes: persistent fatigue, difficulty sleeping, and a growing sense of numbness during client sessions. At first, she told herself she just needed to "push through." But when a client's story triggered an emotional shutdown, Anna realised she couldn't keep ignoring those warning signs.

Reaching out to colleagues and prioritising rest didn't fix everything overnight, but it was the beginning of healing. Anna learned that caring for herself was part of caring for others.

A Note on Healthy Coping Mechanisms

When the cracks start to show, our instinct is often to reach for something—*anything*—to patch them up. And that's completely understandable. We're wired to soothe, to seek relief. But the difference between *numbing out* and *coping well* can be subtle, especially when we're already overwhelmed.

Healthy coping is about finding ways to respond to stress that support your long-term wellbeing, not just mask the symptoms in the short term.

Let's see what this can look like.

Micro-rest for a wired nervous system

Sometimes, rest doesn't mean napping for hours or booking a week off. It starts with five deep breaths between clients, a moment with your hand on your chest, or sitting in the car before you drive home—just breathing, just being. These small pauses give your body a chance to downshift and reset.

Movement without pressure

Forget the gym if it feels like another obligation. What about a short walk while listening to music you loved as a teenager? A few minutes of stretching before bed? Movement can be medicine when it comes from a place of kindness, not punishment.

Journaling that's honest, not polished

You don't have to write beautifully or even make sense. Just letting your feelings spill onto the page—even for ten minutes—can act like an emotional release valve. Try starting with "Right now, I feel..." and see where it goes.

Joy that's bite-sized

Not everything has to be "productive." Watch that ridiculous show. Colour in a children's colouring book. Eat something that makes you feel comforted (just watch that you don't make this a habit!). These tiny joys build emotional resilience. They remind you you're still here, still human, still capable of pleasure.

Support that's reciprocal, not draining

Healthy coping often means connecting with people who get it. Not to vent endlessly (though that can help), but to feel seen and to see others in return. If you don't have that yet, consider a peer support group, a therapist, or a colleague who's walked a similar road.

And most importantly: don't judge your coping mechanisms—just get curious. Are they softening the edges? Or are they stuffing everything down?

You deserve support strategies that *nourish* you, not ones that leave you more depleted.

One important aspect of healthy coping is knowing when to seek professional support. Consulting a qualified health professional can provide clarity, reassurance, and appropriate treatment options— especially when symptoms persist, worsen, or begin to interfere with daily life.

Practical Tips for Spotting and Responding to the Cracks

Tune in daily, even briefly.

Set aside just 5 minutes at the start or end of your day to check in with your body and emotions. Ask yourself: "How am I feeling right now? What is my energy like? Is there tension or worry I'm carrying?" Journaling a sentence or two can help make this a habit.

Honour your need for rest

If your body or mind is whispering "I'm tired," listen. That might mean prioritising sleep, taking a quiet break, or even just sitting still with a warm drink for a few minutes.

Create tiny rituals of self-care

You don't need hours or expensive treatments. It might be as simple as stretching, stepping outside for fresh air, or lighting a candle and breathing deeply. These small acts send a message to yourself that you matter.

Set gentle boundaries

Learning to say "no" or "not right now" is an act of self-respect. Protect your energy by limiting extra tasks or social obligations that drain you.

Reach out for connection

Whether it is a friend, colleague, mentor, or therapist, talking about how you feel can lift some of the weight. Remember, you don't have to carry this alone.

Limit quick fixes

Notice if you are reaching for caffeine, alcohol, or distractions more than usual. These might feel helpful in the moment but often add to exhaustion or numbness.

Practice compassion with yourself

Be as kind to yourself as you would be to a close friend who was struggling. Remind yourself that it is okay to rest, to ask for help, and to take time to heal.

How Are Your Cracks Looking?

Use this simple checklist as a gentle guide. There's no scoring—just notice what feels true for you right now.

Physical:

☐ I feel unusually tired or drained, even after rest.

☐ I'm experiencing headaches, muscle tension, or aches without a clear cause.

☐ My sleep feels restless or insufficient.

☐ I notice digestive issues or lowered immunity.

Emotional:

☐ I feel more irritable or impatient than usual.

☐ I find it hard to feel joy or connection.

☐ I'm feeling emotionally numb or detached.

☐ I experience feelings of hopelessness or overwhelm.

Behavioural:

☐ I'm withdrawing from friends, family, or social activities.

☐ I've started neglecting self-care routines.

☐ I rely more on caffeine, alcohol, or distractions.

☐ I'm struggling to keep up with work or daily tasks.

Cognitive:

☐ I have trouble concentrating or remembering things.

☐ I feel indecisive or overwhelmed by simple choices.

☐ My creativity or problem-solving feels blocked.

☐ I experience "brain fog" or mental fatigue.

If you tick several of these boxes and the feelings or symptoms have lasted for weeks, consider this a gentle nudge to prioritise rest and reach out for support. You deserve care and kindness—from others, but most importantly, from yourself.

Self-Check-In Exercise

Take a quiet moment just for you. Sit or lie down comfortably, and close your eyes or soften your gaze.

Step 1: Ground Yourself. Feel your body supported by the surface beneath you. Notice where you're making contact, and take a slow, gentle breath in... and out.

Step 2: Scan Your Body. Bring your attention to your feet, then slowly move upward through your body— legs, hips, belly, chest, arms, neck, head. Notice any sensations without needing to change them.

Step 3: Name Your Feelings. Ask yourself, "What am I feeling right now—physically and emotionally?" A few simple words are enough.

Step 4: Listen Kindly. Whatever comes up, meet it with compassion. "It's okay to feel this." No fixing— just noticing.

Step 5: Set a Small Intention. Choose one small, kind thing you can do for yourself today—a rest, a walk, a pause. Picture yourself doing it gently. When ready, open your eyes and return to the room.

Simple Mindful Breathing Practice

When you feel overwhelmed or disconnected, your breath is a steady anchor.

Step 1: Notice Your Breath. Sit or lie down, eyes closed if you like. Simply notice your breath without changing it.

Step 2: Breathe In. Inhale slowly through your nose to a count of four. Feel your belly rise.

Step 3: Pause. Hold gently for a count of two.

Step 4: Breathe Out. Exhale through your mouth for a count of six, softening as you do.

Step 5: Repeat. Continue for 4–6 rounds. If your mind wanders, simply guide it back to the breath.

Why This Helps

Mindful breathing calms your nervous system and invites a sense of safety. The self-check-in encourages compassionate awareness, helping you notice your needs before exhaustion takes hold.

Remember: There is no "right" way to feel or breathe. Your breath is your anchor—steady, reliable, and always available.

Chapter 5: How We Got Here

Unpacking the Roots: Why Burnout and Compassion Fatigue Become Our Reality

If burnout and compassion fatigue feel like unwelcome guests that have settled into your life, it is natural to wonder—how did they get here in the first place? What led to this slow unravel? Understanding the "how" is one of the most powerful steps you can take toward healing and change.

This chapter unpacks the layers—personal, professional, and societal—that combine to wear down even the strongest among us. Spoiler: It is rarely just about you.

The Culture of "Always On"

We live in a world that values productivity like a gold standard. The hustle culture, the never-ending to-do lists, the pressure to always be available—these are modern realities that don't pause for breath.

For caregivers and helping professionals, this pressure can be doubled. There's an unspoken expectation to give endlessly without needing much in return. Saying "no" feels almost taboo, and asking for help can feel like admitting weakness.

The Emotional Cost of Caring

Caring for others is often described as a calling. And for many of us in helping professions, that's exactly how it feels—something we're deeply drawn to. But even meaningful, purpose-driven work has an emotional cost.

Every time you bear witness to someone's pain, hold space for their trauma, or offer care in moments of vulnerability, it takes something from you. Over time, the emotional labour accumulates.

This is how **compassion fatigue** develops: a form of emotional and psychological exhaustion caused by the repeated exposure to others' suffering, particularly when there isn't enough time or space to process or recover.

Unlike burnout—which is typically associated with workload, deadlines, and institutional stress—compassion fatigue is about **emotional overload**. It's the weight of being present with suffering, again and again, without enough recovery in between.

You may not even notice it at first. But the signs build:

- You feel numb or emotionally flat when someone shares a difficult story.

- You dread work that used to feel meaningful.

- You snap more easily, or struggle to empathise.

- You come home completely drained, with nothing left for your own family or self.

These are not failures of character. They're predictable outcomes of ongoing emotional strain.

Compassion fatigue is more likely to occur under certain conditions:

High exposure to trauma without support (e.g., in oncology, palliative care, or crisis response)

Minimal debriefing or supervision

Personal trauma history, which may be unconsciously activated

Poor boundaries—such as overextending yourself, not taking breaks, or blurring personal/professional lines

Social conditioning—especially in women and helping professionals, where saying "no" is seen as selfish

Left unaddressed, compassion fatigue can progress to full **burnout**—a deeper, more chronic state that includes emotional exhaustion, depersonalisation, and a diminished sense of accomplishment. At its worst, it can lead to disengagement, physical health issues, and a complete loss of connection to your work and self.

But this trajectory is not inevitable. The first step to healing is recognising what you're carrying—and understanding that it's okay to set it down.

Workload, Resources, and Support

Many of us are working in environments that are **understaffed**, **underfunded**, or missing even the most basic support systems. You might be juggling back-to-back appointments, managing emotional labour on the fly, or taking on extra roles just to keep things running. Long hours, unpredictable rosters, and heavy caseloads are **unsustainable**.

When resources are scarce and demands are high, **burnout becomes a predictable outcome**, not a personal failure.

But even in these challenging environments, there are things we can do—small, strategic shifts that can start to protect your energy and reduce the slow leak of emotional exhaustion.

Solutions That Can Help—Even When Systems Don't

Audit What's Actually in Your Control

When everything feels overwhelming, one of the most powerful things you can do is **separate what's yours to carry** and what isn't. Try this short reflection:

- What tasks drain you most each day?

- What parts of your day feel non-negotiable?

- Are there small things you *can* adjust—even slightly?

Sometimes that means shifting an appointment by 15 minutes so you can breathe, delegating a task (even imperfectly), or saying "no" to an extra obligation without guilt.

Prioritise Micro-Restorative Practices

You may not be able to take a full lunch break every day—but you *can* build in **micro-restorative moments.**
Examples:

- A few slow breaths between clients

- A warm drink away from your screen

- One minute of stretching between tasks

- Journaling for three minutes at the end of your shift

Preserve the part of you that makes the work sustainable.

Advocate Collectively (Not Just Individually)

If possible, connect with peers or colleagues to share the emotional load through regular debriefs. Identify shared issues and bring them to management as a group. You could also create informal peer support circles, even if your workplace doesn't have one.

Even short check-ins ("How are you really doing today?") can make a difference.

Use What's Available

Access to formal supervision, counselling, or mental health support isn't always ideal—but if it *is* available, use it. It doesn't have to be when you're already on the verge of collapse. Prevention is ideal.

If there's no structured support in your workplace, explore:

- Your professional association (some offer free counselling or legal advice)

- Community-run reflective practice groups

- Apps or services that offer trauma-informed peer support (e.g., *Peer Collective*, *TalkLife*, or *Australian Counselling Services*)

Know Your Energy Budget

You wouldn't run your car on empty. You shouldn't run your body that way either. Each week, check in:

- How many clients, hours, or responsibilities can I realistically manage right now?

- What am I saying "yes" to that might need a pause or a boundary?

You are allowed to adjust your capacity based on your current reality—not what the job expects from a machine.

Burnout prevention doesn't always mean changing the whole system (though we'd all love that). Sometimes it starts with protecting one hour, one moment, one part of yourself at a time.

Blurred Line: When Work Follows You Home

For many of us, the physical workday ends—but the emotional work continues long after we've left the building. Whether it's worrying about a client, catching up on notes at the kitchen table, or replaying difficult conversations in our heads while brushing our teeth, the line between "work" and "home" becomes dangerously thin.

Over time, this blurred boundary chips away at your rest, your relationships, and your sense of self.

Strictly enforcing a separation between work and home can serve as a **protective strategy** for your mental health. And in many cases, it's the first step in recognising whether your workplace is genuinely sustainable long-term.

What Might This Look Like in Practice?

Setting non-negotiable stop times. If your shift ends at 5:30, you shut your laptop or walk out the door at 5:30. No "just one more email." Honour that line.

Creating a "transition ritual." A walk, a song, a cup of tea before driving home—something that signals to your brain that work is done. (Yes, even if you work from home.)

Turning off work notifications. That urgent message can wait until morning. You're not on call unless you're *literally* on call.

Communicating your boundaries to management. This part is crucial. You might say:

"I'm noticing I'm not switching off properly after hours, and it's affecting my wellbeing. I'd like to set clearer work/home boundaries so I can show up more fully during work hours."

Being honest with yourself about the bigger picture. For some people, drawing firmer lines brings surprising clarity. If your boundaries are respected, you feel more empowered. If they're not—if pushing back is met with pressure, guilt, or punishment—it may reveal that the environment itself is incompatible with sustainable care.

Personally, once I enforced clear boundaries at work— no out-of-hours tasks, no unpaid emotional labour—I realised something uncomfortable: I was no longer a good fit for that workplace. And that insight, while hard, gave me the permission I needed to leave. The more people recognise and name these patterns, the more pressure we place on employers to build systems that *actually* support those who care for others.

Reflection

How often do you mentally "clock off" when your shift ends?

What does your ideal end-of-work ritual look like?

If you were to have a boundary conversation with your manager, what would you want them to understand?

Personal Factors That Play a Role

Sometimes, our own beliefs and personality traits can contribute. High achievers, perfectionists, and people pleasers are more vulnerable to burnout because of their inner drive and tendency to push beyond limits.

Past experiences, including trauma or unresolved stress, can also increase susceptibility.

Societal and Systemic Contributors

We can't ignore the bigger picture. Societal attitudes toward mental health, lack of adequate healthcare resources, and cultural norms about work and rest shape the environments we live and work in.

For example, stigma around mental health struggles may prevent people from seeking help until things become severe.

Looking Back with Kindness

What cultural or workplace messages about "toughing it out" or "just getting on with it" have influenced how you approach stress and self-care?

Can you identify moments when you pushed past your limits because you felt you "should" or "had to"?

What personal beliefs about your role in caring or working might be contributing to your exhaustion?

How have external factors—like workload, resources, or support—impacted your experience?

What small changes in mindset or environment could begin to shift your experience?

A Story from a Social Worker

Mark had always been proud of the work he did. As a social worker supporting vulnerable families, he saw his role not just as a job, but a calling. He was the one people could rely on—calm in crisis, resourceful under pressure, and always willing to stay late to make sure his clients didn't fall through the cracks.

But the cracks weren't just in the lives of his clients. They were in the system itself.

Mark worked in an agency that was chronically understaffed. Caseloads were high. Deadlines were constant. Every week brought a new emergency. He skipped breaks. Ate lunch in the car. Took phone calls at home. Told himself he could push through— because the people he was helping were worse off. Because he cared.

And he did care. Deeply. But caring without pause or support comes at a cost.

At first, the signs were subtle. He was more tired in the mornings. His concentration slipped. He started forgetting small details—like whether he'd followed up on a referral, or if he'd already returned that call. He brushed it off. Just a busy week.

But the fog didn't lift. He became irritable. Numb. He stopped laughing with his colleagues. His once-patient tone grew flat and transactional. And his clients noticed.

One day, a mother in crisis said quietly,

"You don't look like you care anymore."

That comment stuck in his chest. Not because she was wrong—but because she was right.

Mark's empathy—his greatest strength—had gone quiet. He started dreading work. Each client began to feel like a burden, not a human being. He felt ashamed, like a fraud. He told himself he was failing.

The cascade began:

Because he was emotionally drained, he missed early red flags in cases. Delays followed. Crises escalated. The fallout landed on his teammates—who were already stretched. That, in turn, led to tension in the office, higher stress, more staff turnover. The system frayed, and Mark was at the centre, trying to hold it all together while falling apart himself.

Eventually, he hit a wall. He had a panic attack in the kitchen one morning and couldn't bring himself to go to work. That was the day he realised he couldn't keep going—not like this.

Mark took a leave of absence. At first, he felt like a failure. But with the help of a compassionate GP, a trauma-informed counsellor, and others who had been through the same storm, he began to understand what had really happened. It was about a system designed to reward self-sacrifice—until it breaks the very people it relies on.

Mark was experiencing **compassion fatigue**, **burnout**, and eventually a full **nervous breakdown**—not because he cared too much, but because he had nowhere safe to put that care.

As he recovered, something shifted. Mark began connecting the dots—not just for himself, but for the entire workforce of helpers around him. He started reading, speaking with colleagues, and exploring the **bigger picture**. He realised that unless the *system* changed, more people would fall exactly where he had.

When he was ready, he didn't return to frontline work—but he did return to advocacy. Mark began consulting with organisations on trauma-informed workplace practices. He helped design reflective supervision programs. He trained managers to recognise early signs of burnout in their teams. He spoke honestly about what had happened to him—not with shame, but with clarity.

And slowly, change happened. His former employer introduced protected case review times, more flexible rosters, and mental health support that actually worked. They didn't do it because they suddenly cared more—they did it because people like Mark made it impossible to ignore.

Why This Story Matters

Mark's story is not unusual. What *is* unusual is that he got out—and turned his pain into purpose. Most people stay just long enough to break, then quietly disappear.

But the more we tell these stories, the more we make space for change. When we understand the cost of chronic over-giving— not just to ourselves, but to those we care for—we begin to see boundaries not as walls, but as **acts of advocacy**.

We stop thinking we have to prove our worth through depletion.
We start building a system that allows us to care—and to *keep* caring.

Reflection: Understanding "How We Got Here"

1. Mapping Your Burnout Landscape

Take a blank sheet of paper or your journal. Draw a circle in the middle and write "Me" inside. Around that, draw smaller circles or bubbles representing different factors contributing to your burnout or compassion fatigue. These might include:

- Workload demands

- Emotional strain of caregiving

- Personal beliefs/perfectionism

- Lack of boundaries

- Social or cultural expectations

- Support systems (or lack thereof)

- Physical health

- Sleep and rest habits

Reflect on each bubble: Which feels the heaviest or most draining? Which are within your control to change? Which might need external help?

2. Beliefs Inventory

List three beliefs you hold about yourself or your work that might contribute to pushing yourself too hard. Examples: "I must always be available," "Asking for help is a sign of weakness," or "I'm the only one who can do this well."

For each belief, ask:

- Is this belief true?

- What would I say to a friend?

- How might I reframe this belief to something kinder or more balanced?

3. Timeline Reflection

Think back to when you first noticed signs of burnout or compassion fatigue. Write a short timeline of key moments, feelings, or events that have shaped your experience. This is not about blame but understanding patterns.
Ask yourself:

- Were there turning points or times, I ignored early warning signs?

- What helped me keep going?

- What might I do differently now, with what I know?

Strategies to Start Shifting

1. Set Micro-Boundaries

Start small. For example:

- Turning off work emails for 30 minutes before bed.

- Saying "no" to one extra task this week.

- Scheduling a 10-minute break mid-workday to stretch or breathe.

Micro-boundaries build confidence and show that caring for yourself is not selfish—it is essential.

2. Practice Radical Compassion with Yourself

In a society where kindness is often mistaken for weakness—and where being hard on yourself is seen as a form of discipline—it can feel radical to respond to your own struggles with gentleness. But compassion isn't complacency. It provides clarity. It's strength.

When you notice harsh self-talk or pressure creeping in, try pausing and asking yourself: **"What would I say to a loved one in this moment?"** Then—speak that kindness to yourself, as if you meant it.

This simple shift begins to **rewire your internal dialogue**, soften the weight of expectations, and anchor you in self-compassion that supports—not sabotages—your growth.

Being kind to yourself isn't indulgent. It's essential.

3. Create a Support Map

Identify people, groups, or professionals you can turn to when you need support. This could be a trusted friend, a mentor, a counsellor, or an online community run by professionals. Reach out—even if just to say, "I'm struggling today." Connection is a powerful antidote to isolation.

4. Reclaim Small Joys and Rest

Schedule tiny doses of joy or rest each day—something that feels nourishing but not overwhelming. It might be listening to a favourite song, a quick walk outside, a cup of tea without screens, or a few moments of deep breathing. Or it might be locking the doors, putting the dog outside, securing fragile items, and dancing wildly while singing loudly to a song that makes you feel good. Or it might be going to an art gallery or exhibition, and just being with a piece of art that even mildly "speaks" to you. Experiencing it up close, from afar, and noticing life happening in the periphery of your senses. Whatever it might look like for you, do something that makes you feel good.

5. Advocate for Change and know when to leave

If your work environment contributes to your stress, start a conversation. It could be with a supervisor, HR, or colleagues. Frame it around shared wellbeing: "I think we could all benefit from more regular breaks" or "I'd like to explore ways to better support each other."

Even small changes can ripple outward. If nothing ever changes, you might consider leaving.

6. Mindfulness and Grounding Practices

Incorporate brief mindfulness moments—like the breathing exercise from Chapter 4—to help regulate stress and improve focus. Apps or guided meditations can be helpful if you are new to this.

Closing Thought

Remember, shifting the roots of burnout and compassion fatigue is a marathon, not a sprint. Small, consistent steps build resilience and hope. And you absolutely deserve to feel well—mind, body, and spirit.

Chapter 6: When Helping Becomes Hurting

Boundaries, Blurred Roles, and the Emotional Cost of Over-giving

Experiencing joy from helping others is a gift—a deeply meaningful, often joyful part of our lives. But when the line between helping and hurting becomes fuzzy, the danger is being trapped in a harmful cycle that drains your spirit and energy. You start wondering: *Am I losing myself? Why does caring sometimes feel like a burden?*

This chapter invites you to explore the delicate balance between giving and self-care, to recognize the signs when boundaries are slipping, and to gently reclaim your own space, identity, and wellbeing.

Giver's Guilt: The Invisible Weight

Have you ever wanted to say "no," but felt a sharp pang of guilt that stopped you? That feeling is called *giver's guilt*—a sneaky, invisible weight that ties your sense of worth to how much you can give or sacrifice.

- "If I don't help, who will?"

- "I'm letting people down if I say no."

- "Others need me more than I need rest."

These thoughts come from a place of caring, but they can chain you to a cycle of over-giving. The tricky part is that guilt often feels like a *moral compass*—telling you what a "good person" should do. Guilt can become a barrier to your own wellbeing, slowly eroding your energy and joy.

You are not alone in feeling this. Many caregivers, therapists, nurses, and helpers wrestle with the same invisible burden.

Recognising *giver's guilt* is the first step toward freeing yourself from it.

When We Become the Work

Your work or role—whether professional or personal—can become so intertwined with your identity that it feels impossible to separate. You might hear yourself say, *"This is who I am,"* or *"If I stop doing this, what is left of me?"*

This blurring of self and role is common in caring professions, and whilst it is an extremely positive part of being human, it can also be harmful. When your sense of value is wrapped up in how much you do for others, it is easy to overlook your own needs. Balance what you do for others with what you do for yourself.

Taking a step back to remember *who you are beyond your work*—your passions, quirks, relationships, and dreams—is not just a luxury, but a necessity for sustainable helping.

Over-Responsibility and Loss of Self

The burden of responsibility can be crushing when it is not shared. Feeling responsible for everyone's feelings, success, or happiness is an impossible task—and yet, many helpers fall into this trap.

Over-responsibility can look like:

- Taking on others' emotions as if they were your own.

- Feeling guilty when outcomes are not perfect or beyond your control.

- Believing that you must always be "strong" or "available."

- Sacrificing your own wellbeing to avoid disappointing others.

This mindset can lead to a loss of self, where your own boundaries, desires, and limits become invisible to you. It is like carrying a backpack stuffed with invisible stones—each one a responsibility that weighs you down without others even seeing.

Learning to release the weight of over-responsibility doesn't mean you care less—it means you are realising the importance of balancing the aspects of kindness.

Reflection: Exploring Your Boundaries

Let's explore where your boundaries might be stretched or blurred:

- **Giver's Guilt:** Can you recall a recent time when you felt guilty for putting your needs first? What thoughts or feelings came up?

- **Identity Check:** How much do you feel your role defines your self-worth? What parts of "you" might be getting lost in your work?

- **Boundary Awareness:** Are there moments where you said "yes" but really wanted to say "no"? What held you back?

- **Responsibility Radar:** How much responsibility do you feel for others' emotions or outcomes? Which of these feel fair, and which feel like too much?

- **Vision for Change:** What would a healthier boundary or relationship with responsibility look like for you?

Practical Tips to Reclaim Boundaries and Self

Here are some gentle, practical ways to start reclaiming your boundaries and sense of self:

Tune Into Your Body's Signals

Your body often knows before your mind does. Notice when you feel tension in your shoulders, a tight chest, a racing heart, or apathy creeping in. These signals are your body's way of telling you boundaries might be slipping.

Practice Saying "No" with Compassion

It is okay to say no—and you don't need a big explanation. Try simple phrases like, "I can't take that on right now," or "I need to focus on my own wellbeing today." Saying no is an act of self-respect, not selfishness.

Create Rituals to Mark Transitions

Whether it is changing clothes after work, a short meditation, or a walk around the block, rituals can help your mind and body shift from work mode to personal time, reinforcing healthy boundaries.

Write Down Your Limits

Get clear on what you are willing and able to give. Writing it down helps make boundaries real and easier to communicate.

Ask for Support

Share your boundaries with trusted friends, family, or colleagues. When people understand your limits, they can help respect and reinforce them.

Nurture Your Identity Beyond Work

Reconnect with hobbies, interests, or relationships that bring you joy outside of your caregiving role. This helps remind you there's more to you than your work.

Self-Compassion is Key

When guilt or pressure creeps in, practice self-kindness. Remind yourself that taking care of you is necessary for you to be your best self for others.

A Story to Hold Onto

Emily (not her real name) had always prided herself on being the reliable nurse who "went above and beyond." Over the years, she picked up extra shifts, stayed late to comfort patients, and rarely said no.

But slowly, Emily noticed she was exhausted—not just physically, but emotionally. The joy she once found in her work felt dimmed, replaced by anxiety and a sense of being overwhelmed.

One day, she decided to try something different. She started by setting a simple boundary: no extra shifts without a day off after. She told a me about her struggles and asked for my support in holding her accountable.

Emily also returned to ceramic art — a long-lost passion that filled her with peace. As she nurtured this part of herself, she felt more balanced, more whole.

Setting boundaries wasn't easy at first. The guilt tugged at her. But over time, she realised boundaries were not walls—they were bridges to self-care and sustainable helping.

Reflection: When Helping Becomes Hurting

1. Giver's Guilt Exploration

Think about a recent situation where you wanted to say "no" but said "yes" instead.

What thoughts or feelings were running through your mind at that moment?

Were you afraid of disappointing someone? Feeling selfish? Something else?

How might you reframe those thoughts to be kinder and more realistic?

2. Identity and Role Check-In

Write down the roles or titles you identify with most strongly (e.g., caregiver, therapist, parent, friend).

For each, ask yourself: *How much of my self-worth feels tied to this role?*

What parts of you feel hidden or neglected because of these roles?

How could you make space to nurture those parts of yourself?

3. Boundary Awareness

Recall a time when you felt your boundaries were respected and honoured. What did that feel like?

Now, think of a time when your boundaries were crossed or ignored. How did that impact your wellbeing?

What are some small boundaries you could set this week to protect your energy?

4. Responsibility Reflection

On a scale of 1 to 10, how responsible do you feel for others' emotions or outcomes?

Are there areas where this responsibility feels unfair or overwhelming?

What would it look like to share or release some of that responsibility?

5. Visualising a Healthy Boundary

Close your eyes and imagine a scenario where you successfully set a boundary that felt right for you.

What did you say or do? How did the other person respond?

How did you feel afterward—inside your body and mind?

Write about this experience and how you might bring it into your real life.

6. Self-Compassion Practice

Write a letter to yourself from the perspective of a caring friend who understands your struggles with over-giving.

What would they say to you about guilt, boundaries, and self-care?

How can you show yourself more kindness starting today?

7. Celebrating Small Wins

List three moments in the past week where you respected your own needs or said "no" when you needed to.

Celebrate these wins, no matter how small. How did honouring yourself feel?

Chapter 7: Reclaiming Your Energy

Restoring Balance, Building Resilience, and Finding Joy Again

Burnout and compassion fatigue can leave you feeling empty, drained, and disconnected—not just from your work, but from yourself. The good news is, no matter how tangled or worn out you feel right now, recovery is possible. This chapter invites you to gently reclaim your energy, restore balance in your life, and find your way back to joy and meaning.

The Power of Rest and Renewal

We live in a culture that often glorifies constant doing—nonstop work, relentless productivity, endless giving. But rest is not the enemy of success or care; it is the foundation. Rest is what replenishes your body, mind, and soul so you can continue to give authentically without losing yourself.

Rest looks different for everyone. For some, it might be a deep sleep or a lazy weekend morning. For others, it is quiet moments of meditation or journaling. It might even be a short walk outside, breathing fresh air and feeling grounded.

Giving yourself permission to rest is a radical act of self-compassion. It is saying: *I am worthy of care. My needs matter.* Rest is not indulgence; it is essential.

If rest has been missing in your life, start small. Notice when your body signals fatigue or stress. Maybe it is a tight jaw, a headache, or difficulty focusing. These signals are your body's way of asking for a break. Listen kindly, and give yourself what you need—even if it is just five minutes of mindful breathing.

Building Resilience Without Burning Out

Resilience is often misunderstood as "toughing it out," but real resilience is more about flexibility, self-awareness, and smart self-care. It means adapting to challenges without losing your sense of self or wellbeing.

Here are some ways to build resilience that supports long-term wellbeing:

Create daily routines that nurture you. This might include morning stretches, mindful eating, or evening gratitude practices. These small habits build emotional reserves.

Stay connected. Healthy relationships—whether friends, family, or colleagues—provide support and remind you that you are not alone.

Set realistic goals. Break big tasks into manageable steps, and celebrate progress, not perfection.

Practice self-compassion. When you stumble or feel overwhelmed, treat yourself like a dear friend rather than a harsh critic.

Remember, resilience is not about avoiding stress or challenges but learning how to recover from them with kindness and wisdom.

Finding Joy and Meaning Again

When burnout seeps in, it can dull your sense of purpose and joy. But these can be reclaimed—and often, in surprising ways.

At the same time, allow yourself to explore new sources of joy and meaning outside your work. Maybe it is a hobby you set aside, a creative project, or simply spending time with loved ones without agenda.

Joy is not frivolous; it is fuel. It replenishes your spirit and makes the work sustainable.

Reflection

What recent moments, no matter how small, have brought you peace or happiness?

How can you invite more of these moments into your life regularly?

Who in your life provides you with genuine support? How can you nurture those connections?

What is one small daily habit you can start to protect your energy and wellbeing?

How can you practice kindness toward yourself when things feel overwhelming?

Mindful Energy Check-In

Pause for a moment and check in with your energy.

- Find a comfortable seated position and close your eyes.
- Take three slow, deep breaths, noticing the air filling your lungs and slowly leaving your body.

- Scan your body from head to toe. Notice where you feel tension, heaviness, or lightness. Don't judge—just observe.
- Ask yourself: *What would make me feel more balanced? Rest? Movement? Connection?*
- Commit to one small action today that honours that need.

Reclaiming your energy is about learning to dance with life's challenges with grace, to honour your limits, and to nurture the vibrant person you are beneath the caregiving role.

You deserve to feel whole, joyful, and alive—and taking care of yourself is the first step to that beautiful reclamation.

Chapter 8: The Healing Journey

From Awareness to Action — Moving Forward with Hope and Intention

Healing is not only possible, but also within your reach. The path to recovery may be winding, and it won't always be easy, but it can lead to a deeper connection with yourself, renewed energy, and a more balanced, fulfilling way of living and caring.

This chapter is an invitation to step gently from awareness into action — to begin crafting your own healing journey, one small step at a time, rooted in kindness, patience, and hope.

Embracing Awareness as a Catalyst for Change

The moment you recognize that burnout or compassion fatigue has taken hold is a powerful and turning point. Awareness is like shining a gentle, curious light into the corners of your experience that might have felt hidden or overwhelming. It opens the door to new possibilities.

This awareness is not a sign of failure or weakness—it is a gift. It shows that you are ready to listen to your needs and honour your limits. Healing begins with compassion for where you are right now, exactly as you are. You might feel tired, frustrated, or scared, and that's okay. You are not alone in this, and these feelings are part of the process.

It is important to acknowledge that healing is rarely linear. Some days you will make progress; others you'll feel like you don't. Both are normal. What matters most is the ongoing intention to care for yourself and move forward gently.

Crafting Your Healing Plan

Healing is deeply personal. What works for one person may not work for another, and that's why your healing plan needs to be tailored to your unique situation, preferences, and strengths. There's no one-size-fits-all solution—only what feels right and manageable for you.

Here are some foundational elements to consider including in your plan:

Restorative Practices: These might be activities that soothe your body and mind, such as meditation, yoga, tai chi, gentle stretching, or spending time in nature. Creative outlets like painting, writing, or music can also be deeply healing. Even simple pleasures like a warm bath or listening to your favourite music count as restorative.

Social Connection: Isolation often deepens burnout, so cultivating meaningful connections is crucial. This could mean reaching out to trusted friends, joining a support group, or talking with peers who understand your experience. Sharing your story and hearing others' can reduce feelings of loneliness and foster hope.

Professional Support: Sometimes, healing requires additional help from trained professionals such as therapists, counsellors, or coaches. Seeking support is a brave step and can provide you with tools and perspectives to navigate your journey more effectively.

Boundary Setting: Learning to say "no" and protect your time and energy is vital. This might mean setting limits on work hours, social commitments, or emotional availability. Remember, boundaries are acts of self-respect, not selfishness.

Self-Compassion Rituals: Develop daily or weekly habits that nurture your inner dialogue. This could be journaling, practicing affirmations, or simply pausing to check in with yourself. Treat yourself as kindly as you would a beloved friend.

Start with small, achievable steps rather than trying to overhaul everything at once. Each positive change, no matter how minor it seems, builds momentum and fosters resilience.

Staying Open to Growth and Change

Healing often asks us to release old patterns, beliefs, and habits that no longer serve us. This can be uncomfortable or even frightening because it means stepping into the unknown.

However, this openness can also be deeply liberating. You may find yourself rediscovering forgotten parts of yourself—your creativity, your curiosity, your laughter. Healing can lead you to new passions or ways of living that better align with your values and needs.

For some, this might mean rethinking their role in caregiving or their career path altogether. For others, it might simply mean finding better balance and healthier ways to engage.

Growth is not about perfection. It is about embracing imperfection, learning from mistakes, and moving forward with compassion.

Reflection

What does healing look like and feel like to you? Try to describe it in as much detail as possible.

What is one small step you feel ready to take today to nurture yourself?

Who in your life can you turn to for support? How can you reach out to them?

How can you practice patience with yourself during this process, especially when progress feels slow?

What old beliefs or habits might you be willing to release to make space for healing and growth?

What new possibilities or interests are you curious about exploring?

Creating a Healing Map

A Healing Map is a personalised, visual guide to your journey. It helps you clarify your needs, resources, and goals in a way that's easy to revisit and update.

How to create your Healing Map:

1. Grab a large sheet of paper or a journal.

2. In the center, write "My Healing Journey" or a phrase that feels meaningful to you.

3. Around the center, draw or list:

- Areas of your life needing attention or care (e.g. sleep, relationships, work balance).
- Resources and people who support you (e.g. friends, therapists, hobbies).
- Practices that bring you peace or joy (e.g. meditation, walking, reading).
- Signs that show you are making progress (e.g. better sleep, feeling calmer).

4. Decorate your map with colours, symbols, or drawings that inspire you.

5. Place your Healing Map somewhere visible as a reminder of your commitment to yourself.

Return to this map regularly, updating it as you grow and change.

Final Thoughts

Healing from burnout and compassion fatigue is not a destination but a lifelong journey. It requires patience, kindness, and persistence. You might stumble, but each time you rise with care for yourself, you grow stronger.

This journey can transform your pain into wisdom, your exhaustion into resilience, and your struggle into a deeper, more compassionate connection with yourself and others.

You are worthy of healing. You are deserving of rest, joy, and balance. And you have everything within you to reclaim your energy and thrive once again.

Tools and Support for Your Healing Journey

Books and Reading

"Burnout: The Secret to Unlocking the Stress Cycle" by Emily Nagoski and Amelia Nagoski
A compassionate and science-backed guide that explains how stress affects the body and offers practical tools to complete the stress cycle and build resilience.

"The Gifts of Imperfection" by Brené Brown
A warm invitation to embrace your imperfections, cultivate self-compassion, and live wholeheartedly.

"Radical Acceptance" by Tara Brach
A beautiful exploration of mindfulness and self-compassion as paths to healing and freedom.

"Compassion Fatigue Workbook: Creative Tools for Transforming Compassion Fatigue and Vicarious Traumatization" by Francoise Mathieu
This workbook offers practical exercises designed

specifically for caregivers and helpers facing compassion fatigue.

Websites and Online Communities

Compassion Fatigue Awareness Project
compassionfatigue.org

A hub for education, support, and resources for those struggling with compassion fatigue.

The Center for Mindful Self-Compassion
self-compassion.org

Offers free resources, guided meditations, and training programs on cultivating self-compassion.

Headspace
headspace.com

An app with guided mindfulness and meditation practices—perfect for beginners and seasoned practitioners alike.

Burnout Australia
burnout.org.au

Australian-based resources and support for burnout prevention and recovery.

Practical Tools and Apps

Insight Timer (Free app)
Offers thousands of free guided meditations focused on stress, sleep, compassion, and self-care.

Moodfit (Free and paid versions)
A mood-tracking app with tools for managing stress, sleep, and mental wellbeing.

Calm (Subscription-based app)
Guided meditations, breathing exercises, and sleep stories designed to reduce anxiety and improve sleep quality.

Professional Support and Networks

Find a Mental Health Professional

In Australia, search for a psychologist or counsellor through **Better Access** (via Medicare) or private providers through the **Australian Psychological Society** at psychology.org.au.

Employee Assistance Programs (EAP)

Many workplaces offer free confidential counselling services through EAPs—check with your employer.

Peer Support Groups

Look for local or online peer support groups focused on caregiver wellbeing, burnout recovery, or specific professions (healthcare, social work, therapy).

Self-Care and Boundary Setting Resources

Books:

"Boundaries: When to Say Yes, How to Say No To Take Control of Your Life" by Dr. Henry Cloud and Dr. John Townsend

"The Art of Extreme Self-Care" by Cheryl Richardson

Articles and Guides:

MindTools: Setting Boundaries [mindtools.com/pages/article/newTCS_98.htm]

Verywell Mind: How to Set Healthy Boundaries [verywellmind.com/how-to-set-boundaries-5079472]

Gentle Reminders

Healing takes time — be patient and gentle with yourself.

Small, consistent self-care practices often have the biggest impact.

Reaching out for help is a sign of strength, not weakness.

You deserve rest, joy, and renewal.

Chapter 9: The Myth of Quick Fixes

Why Bubble Baths and Gratitude Journals Are Not Enough

If you've ever felt overwhelmed by burnout or compassion fatigue, you might have tried the classic "quick fixes": a bubble bath, a gratitude journal, a mindfulness app, or a weekend off. While these are lovely and certainly helpful in small doses, the truth is that real recovery runs much deeper.

This chapter peels back the myth that simple, surface-level fixes can undo the complex web of exhaustion, emotional depletion, and systemic stress. We explore why "self-care" can sometimes feel like a band-aid on a broken bone, and why rest—true rest—is a radical and revolutionary act.

The Problem with "Self-Care" as a Prescription

The wellness industry has flooded us with ideas of self-care that often feel like just another task on a never-ending to-do list. When we're burned out, being told to "just practice more self-care" can come across as dismissive or even shaming. It can leave us feeling like we're failing if we don't journal daily or meditate for 20 minutes every morning.

Caring for yourself is about deeply tuning in to the needs of your body, mind, and spirit. And often, that means acknowledging limits, saying no, and creating space—not adding more.

Surface Strategies versus Systemic Healing

Bubble baths soothe muscles, and gratitude journals can shift mindset, but they are surface strategies. They may provide temporary relief but don't address underlying causes such as:

- Overwork or unrealistic expectations

- Lack of boundaries in personal and professional life

- Chronic stressors that are structural or systemic

- Emotional labour without adequate support

Systemic healing means addressing these root causes, which often requires changes beyond the individual level: workplace culture, social support, and how we relate to ourselves.

Rest as a Radical Act

In a culture that prizes productivity and "doing," choosing rest is revolutionary. Rest is not just sleep or a day off—it is a radical reclamation of your right to pause, breathe, and restore.

Rest can take many forms: quiet moments of stillness, creative play, time spent in nature, simply saying no to obligations. It is an essential foundation for healing burnout and compassion fatigue.

Rest is not laziness. It is resistance to burnout and a profound act of self-respect.

The Quiet Power of the Arts in Healing

In the noise and urgency of burnout recovery, one form of rest is often overlooked: the kind that happens when we create. When we draw, paint, write, sing, or dance—not for anyone else, not to be productive, but simply to reconnect with something tender and true inside ourselves.

Creative expression is not just a hobby or a luxury. It is a form of self-care, nervous system regulation, and even identity repair.

In fact, numerous studies confirm what many of us already know instinctively:

- A 2016 study in *Art Therapy: Journal of the American Art Therapy Association* found that engaging in just **45 minutes of creative activity** significantly reduced cortisol levels (the stress hormone) in adults, regardless of artistic experience.

- Research published in *Frontiers in Psychology* (2019) highlighted that **art-making promotes psychological resilience**, emotional processing, and restoration—especially in those experiencing occupational stress or trauma exposure.

- Music therapy, creative writing, and visual arts are now widely used in clinical settings for treating **anxiety, PTSD, depression**, and chronic stress-related conditions (Stuckey & Nobel, 2010; Bolwerk et al., 2014).

But you don't need a research paper to know that sitting down with a blank page, humming to a favourite song, or crafting something with your hands can feel like an exhale.

When the work you do involves holding space for others, the arts allow you to hold space for yourself— not by fixing anything, but by **making meaning** from the mess. They help you process what you can't put into words. They remind you that you are more than your role, your responsibilities, your exhaustion.

You don't need to be "good" at art. You just need to be present. Let go of outcomes. Create badly, joyfully, honestly. That's where the magic is.

Try this:

- Doodle for 5 minutes with no plan.

- Journal with the prompt "Right now, I feel..." and write without editing.

- Play a piece of music that makes you feel something and move your body—no choreography required.

- Try blackout poetry: take an old book page or newspaper and black out words to form a poem.

- Make a collage of images that feel like *you*.

The arts reconnect you to your *aliveness*. And sometimes, that's the most radical form of healing of all. The arts provide profound perspectives of ourselves (as a community and an individual), in relation to the outside world. A sense of being part of something much larger than ourselves.

Sometimes it can be a common thread within a work of art that makes you realise you're not alone in feeling the way you do.

Other times it can open up and inspire new ideas you might not have otherwise thought of.

Art can bring joy and perspective.

You can also just enjoy art by reading a good book, listening to some quiet music, or experiencing an art exhibition.

Art can also be realising the beauty of the negative space between the branches of a tree that lets the sunlight through, or the ripples in the sand the waves leave behind.

Appreciating art is being with the joy and beauty in the world.

Reflection

When has "self-care" felt helpful, and when has it felt like another chore?

What parts of your life contribute to your exhaustion that surface self-care can't fix?

What would radical rest look like for you?

How can you begin to set boundaries that support systemic healing?

Practical Exercise: Designing Your Radical Rest Plan

Take time to identify what true rest means for you beyond the usual quick fixes. Consider:

- What activities or environments restore your energy?

- What obligations can you pause or reduce to create space?

- How will you protect your rest time from interruption or guilt?

Create a simple plan for incorporating radical rest into your routine—even if it is just 5 minutes a day to start.

Chapter 10: Reclaiming Rest and Rhythm

Recovering from burnout and compassion fatigue is about reconnecting—with ourselves, our bodies, and the natural rhythms that sustain us. It means learning to rest in a way that truly restores and discovering the pace that feels right for *you*.

Let's walk through what real rest looks like, how to spot when we're just distracting ourselves, and how to gently tune into our own unique rhythm. We will also explore the amazing role our nervous system plays in healing and how small, nurturing practices can make a big difference.

Real Rest versus Numbing Out

Have you ever found yourself binge-watching TV or endlessly scrolling on your phone, only to feel just as exhausted or anxious afterward? That's what I mean by "numbing out." It might feel like rest in the moment, but it doesn't give your body or mind the real break it desperately needs.

Real rest is different. It is deep and intentional. It lets your body soften and your mind quiet. It is the kind of rest that helps your muscles relax, your heart rate slow, and your stress hormones ease. This kind of rest invites your nervous system into a state of calm and safety, what science calls the "parasympathetic" state (Porges, 2011).

So, while that bubble bath or gratitude journal can be lovely, true rest goes beyond these quick comforts.

Finding Your Personal Pace

One of the most freeing parts of recovery is realizing there's no one-size-fits-all schedule for rest and activity. We each have a unique rhythm, a personal cadence that's shaped by our bodies, minds, and life stories.

Maybe you notice mornings are your power time, when ideas flow and energies feel high. Or perhaps evenings bring you a quiet calm perfect for gentle reflection. The key is paying attention—and trusting what you learn.

Life often pushes us to hustle non-stop, but honouring your natural pace can be a radical act of self-love. It helps protect you from the exhaustion of constantly running on someone else's clock (Roenneberg, 2019).

Try noticing: When do you feel truly alive? When does your energy dip? How can you arrange your day to ride those waves instead of fighting them?

The Nervous System and Recovery

Our nervous system is the unsung hero in healing from burnout. When we're stressed or overwhelmed, it is often stuck in "fight, flight, or freeze" mode—our bodies on high alert, ready to react but never fully able to relax.

Dr. Stephen Porges' Polyvagal Theory helps us understand how our nervous system moves between states of stress and safety (Porges, 2011). True recovery happens when we can gently shift ourselves back into that safe, calm space where the body knows it is okay to rest and heal.

We can support this shift with simple, loving practices:

Slow, deep breathing: Even a few mindful breaths can calm your heart and ease tension (Lehrer et al., 2020).

Gentle movement: A slow walk, stretching, or yoga reconnects you with your body and invites relaxation (Field, 2016).

Mindfulness: Paying kind attention to the present moment helps quiet racing thoughts and soothe anxiety (Kabat-Zinn, 2005).

Connection: Spending time with people who see and support you reminds your nervous system it is safe to let down your guard (Cacioppo & Patrick, 2008).

These small acts add up, helping you rebuild your energy and resilience from the inside out.

Reflection

Think about your recent days. When did you feel truly rested? When were you just distracting yourself? How did each feel afterward?

What rhythms have you noticed in your energy and mood? How might you lean into those more gently?

Who or what makes you feel safe and cared for? How can you invite more of that into your life?

When did you last notice your breath slowing down naturally? How might you bring that softness into your day?

Practical Exercises

Nervous System Check-In

Find a comfortable spot, close your eyes if you like, and take three slow, full breaths. Notice where you feel tightness or ease in your body. Name one small, kind thing you can do for yourself in this moment—a stretch, a few breaths, a sip of water.

Rhythm Mapping

Over the next few days, jot down your energy levels morning, afternoon, and evening. Notice patterns— when do you feel most alive? When do you need to slow down? Use this insight to plan your day around your natural rhythm, not a clock set by someone else.

Chapter 11: Rebuilding Boundaries (Without Feeling Like a Monster)

Practical Boundaries for Compassionate People

If you are someone who cares deeply—about your clients, your family, your friends—it is easy to feel like boundaries are a betrayal. Maybe you worry that saying no will make you seem selfish, uncaring, or even "like a monster." I want you to know: setting boundaries is one of the kindest things you can do— for yourself and for others.

Boundaries are not walls built to shut people out. They're the gentle fences that keep your energy safe and allow you to show up fully and sustainably. They create the space for authentic connection and compassion to grow, not shrink.

Why Compassionate People need Boundaries

When we care, we tend to give and give—sometimes until there's nothing left. But over-giving leads to exhaustion, resentment, and sometimes burnout. Boundaries help you protect your emotional and physical resources so that your compassion remains a gift, not a drain.

Scripts, Scaffolds, and Baby Steps

Boundaries can feel tricky at first—especially if you've spent years putting others first. The good news? You don't have to leap into that big, bold "no" right away. Start small.

Scripts can help take the guesswork out of setting limits. Here are a few gentle ways to say no or set a boundary:

- "I'm honoured you asked, but I won't be able to give this the attention it deserves right now."

- "Thank you for understanding that I need to prioritize my wellbeing today."

- "I'm unable to help with that, but I'm happy to support you in other ways."

Scaffolding means building support around yourself—like reminders, accountability buddies, or journaling about your feelings. It helps you practice boundaries until they feel more natural.

Saying No Without Guilt

Guilt is one of the biggest hurdles in boundary-setting. But guilt often comes from confusing kindness with self-sacrifice. Saying no doesn't mean you are uncaring—it means you are caring *enough* to protect your health.

When guilt pops up, try this:

- Pause and breathe.

- Remind yourself that your needs are valid.

- Remember that by caring for yourself, you can better care for others.

It is okay to be imperfect. It is okay to say no. It is okay to choose you.

Boundaries as Love, Not Punishment

Think of boundaries as acts of love—not punishment or rejection. When you set a boundary, you are loving yourself enough to say, "I deserve respect and care."

You are also inviting others to love and respect you in return.

Boundaries teach others how to treat you. They create healthier, clearer relationships where everyone's needs can be honoured.

Reflection

What is one area in your life where boundaries feel especially hard? Why?

What small boundary could you practice this week? How might you gently communicate it?

When have you said no in the past and felt relief or freedom afterward? What helped?

How can you remind yourself that setting boundaries is an act of love and self-respect?

Baby Steps to Boundaries

1. Identify one situation this week where you feel stretched too thin or uncomfortable.

2. Choose one small boundary to try—for example, limiting time on calls, saying no to an extra task, or asking for a break.

3. Write down a simple script you can use to express your boundary kindly.

4. Afterward, journal how it felt. What went well? What was challenging?

5. Celebrate your courage—each step forward strengthens your boundary muscles.

Setting boundaries doesn't make you a monster. It makes you human—and it is one of the bravest, kindest things you can do for yourself and those you care about.

Here are some realistic, warm, and practical scripts for common boundary-setting scenarios that feel natural—no corporate speak or robotic phrases here. These are designed to help compassionate people say no or set limits without feeling awkward or harsh.

Scripts for Common Boundary Scenarios

When someone asks for help, but you are already overwhelmed

"Thanks for thinking of me! I'm not able to take that on right now, but I'm here to support you in other ways if I can."

When you need to leave work on time or take a break

"I've got to wrap up at [time] today to take care of some personal things—thanks for understanding."

"I'm going to step away for a bit to recharge. I will be back feeling refreshed and ready to help."

When someone's behaviour or words feel hurtful or draining

"I care about you, but this topic is tough for me at the moment. Can we pause and revisit it later?"

When asked to do something that's outside your role or comfort zone

"I'm not the best person for that, but I can help you find someone who is."

When someone expects immediate replies or constant availability

"I've set some boundaries around my work hours, so I might not respond right away, but I will get back to you as soon as I can."

"I'm offline during evenings to rest and recharge—thanks for understanding."

When you want to decline a social invitation without hurting feelings

"Thanks for thinking of me. I need some downtime, but I'd love to catch up another time."

Remember that saying "NO" is a complete sentence. You really don't have to justify yourself.

I believe it's far tougher to say no after you've already said yes, but it's often much easier to begin with no and then choose to say yes.

Tips for Using Scripts

- Keep your tone warm and honest. You don't need to over-explain—simple is often kinder.

- Remember: you are allowed to put your needs first.

- You don't owe anyone justification—your well-being is reason enough.

Chapter 12: Remembering Who You Are

Reconnection, Redefinition, and Rediscovery

When burnout and compassion fatigue have crept into your life, it can feel like you've lost pieces of yourself along the way. The roles you play—the caregiver, the helper, the therapist, the partner—may have started to define you so completely that you barely recognize the person underneath.

But here's the hopeful truth: deep inside, you are still there. Your core self—the values, passions, and unique spark that make you *you*—is waiting patiently to be remembered, redefined, and rediscovered.

This chapter is an invitation to gently peel back the layers, reconnect with what truly matters, and begin to envision a version of yourself that feels whole and alive again.

Reconnection: Coming Home to Yourself

Recovery begins with coming home to yourself. This means tuning into your feelings, needs, and dreams— without judgment or pressure. It is about listening deeply to the quiet voice beneath the noise of exhaustion and obligation.

You might find this in small moments: savouring your morning coffee, noticing the way sunlight feels on your skin, or remembering a hobby that once brought you joy.

Reconnection is the first step to reclaiming your life, reminding yourself that you are *more* than the burnout and fatigue.

Redefinition: Shaping a New Story

When you've been worn down by endless giving, your identity can feel tangled in the expectations of others. Redefinition is about gently untangling those threads and choosing which parts of your story you want to carry forward—and which ones you are ready to let go.

This might mean redefining what success, worth, and contribution look like for *you*, not anyone else. It is about setting new intentions that align with your values and authentic self, even if they don't match old patterns.

Rediscovery: Joy and Meaningful Work

Rediscovery is the exciting part—exploring what truly lights you up, what gives your life meaning beyond the roles you've been playing. This might be a creative pursuit, a new career direction, deeper relationships, or simply reclaiming a sense of playfulness and curiosity.

Many people find that healing opens doors to a richer, more nuanced sense of purpose—one that honours their limits and celebrates their strengths.

Identity Beyond Roles

Who are you if you are not the helper, the healer, or the "strong one"? This question can feel scary but also freeing.

Your identity is multi-layered and ever evolving. It includes your values, passions, quirks, and dreams. It includes your stories of struggle and resilience. It is who you are when no one is watching.

Allow yourself space to explore this broader identity, free from judgment or pressure to "perform."

What Healing Might Look Like

Healing is not a linear path or a neat destination. It is a journey with twists, turns, and unexpected discoveries. Sometimes it feels like two steps forward and one step back—and that's okay.

Healing might look like small daily rituals that nurture your soul, seeking support when needed, or saying no to what no longer serves you.

It might also look like rediscovering joy in simple pleasures, reconnecting with loved ones, or embracing new possibilities.

Remember: healing is uniquely yours. It honours your pace, your pain, and your potential.

Reflection

What parts of yourself have you lost touch with during burnout or compassion fatigue?

What values or passions feel most important to you right now?

How might you redefine success or fulfillment in a way that feels true to you?

What small step could you take today to reconnect with joy or meaning?

Who are you beneath your roles and responsibilities?

Exercises for Rediscovering Values and Self

Values Reflection Exercise

Take a quiet moment and write down the values that truly matter to you—those guiding principles that feel like your inner compass. Here are some prompts to get you started:

- What qualities do you admire most in others?

- When have you felt most fulfilled or proud of yourself?

- What do you want to stand for, no matter what?

Try to narrow your list down to 3–5 core values. These are the roots that can ground you as you rebuild your life.

Joy Inventory

List activities, moments, or experiences that bring you hoy. It could be as simple as:

- Listening to your favourite song

- Walking barefoot on grass or sand

- Cooking a meal you love

- Talking with a friend who makes you laugh

Keep this list handy and revisit it when you need a reminder of what lights you up.

Identity Mapping

Draw a circle in the middle of a page and write "Me" inside it. Around this circle, jot down words, roles, interests, feelings, or descriptions that make up your identity beyond your work or caregiving role. For example:

- Sister

- Lover of nature

- Curious learner

- Kind-hearted but strong

This visual can help you see the richness of who you are.

Future Self Letter

Write a letter to your future self, imagining where you want to be emotionally and spiritually six months or a year from now. What advice, encouragement, or reminders would you give? What dreams or hopes do you want to nurture?

"Rest and self-care are so important. When you take time to replenish your spirit, it allows you to serve others from the overflow."

— Oprah Winfrey

"Healing takes courage, and we all have courage, even if we have to dig a little to find it."

— Tori Amos

Chapter 13: The Ongoing Journey

Burnout Recovery Isn't Linear—And That's Okay

If you've made it this far, congratulations. You are here, reading these words, ready to keep moving forward on a path that's uniquely yours.

One of the most important truths to embrace is this: recovery from burnout and compassion fatigue is not a straight, predictable road. It is a winding journey full of ups, downs, and unexpected turns. Sometimes you'll feel like you are making great progress, and other times it may seem like you are slipping back into old patterns.

And you know what? That's perfectly okay.

Relapse and Recalibration: The Gentle Art of Course Correction

Many people fear relapse as if it means failure or weakness. But relapse—those moments when exhaustion or overwhelm return—is a natural part of healing. It is a reminder that you are human and that healing is ongoing.

Relapse often happens because life's demands shift suddenly, or because the strategies you've been using need refreshing. Maybe a deadline piled on extra pressure, or a personal challenge demanded more of your emotional reserves. Whatever the trigger, the important thing is what you do next.

This is where recalibration comes in. Recalibration is the compassionate pause that allows you to check in with yourself honestly. What is working? What is not? Which boundaries have weakened? Which self-care practices have been neglected?

It is not about beating yourself up for "slipping." Instead, it is about gentle curiosity and kindness— acknowledging where you are without judgment, and making small adjustments to your habits, routines, or mindset.

For example, if you notice your evenings filled with work emails again, maybe it is time to reinstate a no-work-after-7pm rule. Or if you've stopped your regular walks, perhaps it is time to reclaim that ritual, even if just for 10 minutes a day.

Recalibration is a powerful act of self-respect. It is saying to yourself, "I see you. I'm here with you. Let's find a better way forward together."

What Thriving Really Looks Like

It is easy to imagine thriving as some grand, perfect state of unshakeable happiness or boundless energy. But thriving is more subtle—and far more real.

Thriving means living a life where you have the tools, supports, and habits that allow you to recover more quickly when stress hits, to feel connected to your purpose, and to experience moments of joy even amid challenges.

It might look like:

- Starting your day with a simple grounding ritual—maybe a few mindful breaths or a cup of tea savoured slowly—that centres and calms you.

- Feeling empowered to say "no" without guilt or apology when your limits are reached.

- Having a trusted circle of friends, mentors, or therapists you can turn to when you need emotional support.

- Finding pockets of joy in everyday things: a laugh with a colleague, a song that makes you dance, a quiet moment in nature.

- Accepting that imperfection is part of being human and allowing yourself grace when things are not perfect.

Thriving is not about being invincible. It is about building resilience—the ability to bend without breaking, to recover without shame, and to keep moving forward with compassion for yourself.

A More Sustainable Kind of Care: The Heart of the Matter

If you are someone who gives a lot—whether as a therapist, caregiver, parent, or friend—you might have thought the answer to burnout was simply to "give more" or "try harder."

But the truth is the opposite.

The most sustainable, life-giving kind of care is one that begins with you. It starts with honouring your needs, acknowledging your limits, and making your wellbeing a priority.

This means:

- Setting clear boundaries that protect your energy rather than drain it.

- Saying "no" sometimes, even when it feels uncomfortable, because your "Yes.", must be meaningful.

- Recognizing that self-care is not a luxury or a one-off bubble bath—it is a daily commitment to nurture yourself physically, emotionally, and spiritually.

- Allowing yourself to ask for help and accept support without guilt.

- Being gentle with yourself when you stumble, knowing that healing is messy and imperfect.

This kind of care is not selfish. It is revolutionary. When you care for yourself well, you can show up more fully for others, not out of obligation or depletion, but from a place of genuine presence and generosity.

Moving Forward: Your Ongoing Journey

Remember: this book is not a manual that magically fixes everything overnight. It is a companion on your ongoing journey—one that requires patience, self-awareness, and kindness.

Recovery is about progress, not perfection. There will be days when you feel energized and hopeful, and days when you feel weary and uncertain. Both are part of the process.

So, give yourself permission to move at your own pace. Celebrate small wins. Reach out when you need support. Practice self-compassion like it is your most vital medicine—because it is.

As you continue this journey, hold onto the knowledge that you are more than your burnout, more than your compassion fatigue. You are a whole, evolving person, capable of healing, growth, and thriving.

Compassion with a Backbone: Activism as a Form of Recovery

Many people who burn out do so not because they don't care—but because they care **so much**. They see injustice. They feel suffering. And they're frustrated by how often systems fail the people they were supposed to help.

That anger, that heartbreak, that sense of injustice? It doesn't need to be extinguished—it can be **reclaimed** and **redirected**.

For some, part of recovering from compassion fatigue includes reconnecting with **values-based action.** That might mean:

- **Advocating for fairer workplace practices**

- **Joining campaigns for better mental health access or carer support**

- **Educating others about inequality, ableism, trauma, or healthcare systems**

- **Supporting grassroots efforts for climate, social, or economic justice**

This is not about martyrdom or burnout. This is about **conscious, sustainable activism**—action that aligns with your values *without costing your wellbeing.*

When done in community and with clear boundaries, this kind of involvement can be *energising.* It provides:

- A sense of purpose beyond the daily grind

- Connection with others who care deeply

- A healthy outlet for frustration and grief

- The chance to be part of something bigger

Research supports this too: studies in social psychology and occupational health (e.g., Klar &

Kasser, 2009; Hope et al., 2019) show that **engagement in values-aligned activism can increase wellbeing**, life satisfaction, and resilience—especially when accompanied by emotional support and clear role boundaries.

So yes, tick that social wellness box. But more than that: let your compassion stretch beyond individual care and into collective care.

The goal here is to care *better*. To channel your energy into work that sustains you, and that slowly, steadily, bends the world a little closer to what it should be.

Reflection

When have you noticed signs that you need to pause or slow down? What helped you in those moments?

What are some warning signs you can watch for that suggest it is time to recalibrate?

Who can you reach out to when you need support, and how might you strengthen those connections?

What small, nourishing rituals help you feel grounded and cared for?

How do you want to redefine what thriving means for you personally?

What message of kindness can you offer yourself when the road feels hard?

Practical Strategies for Staying Balanced

Daily check-in: Take five minutes each day to ask yourself, "How am I feeling right now? What do I need?" Write down your answer or simply note it mentally. Use this as a guide to adjust your day.

Support map: Make a list of people, groups, or resources you can turn to in times of stress or overwhelm. Include friends, family, professionals, or even online communities.

Boundary refresh: Review your boundaries regularly. Are they working? Do they need tweaking? Remember, boundaries are living things that can change as your needs evolve.

Self-compassion practice: When you catch yourself in negative self-talk or guilt, pause and ask, "Would I say this to a dear friend? How can I be kinder to myself?"

Chapter 14: For the Therapist, the Healer, the Human

Final Reflections for Those Who Hold Space for Others

To you who hold the space—the therapist, the healer, the human—this chapter is written with deep gratitude and tenderness.

You are the quiet strength behind so many transformations, the steady presence in moments of vulnerability, the compassionate heart that offers safety in uncertainty.

Yet, beneath this noble calling lies a truth too often hidden: you are human, too. You carry your own fears, wounds, hopes, and fatigue. The very act of holding space for others can sometimes leave your own heart feeling empty, your spirit tired.

This chapter is your sanctuary—a place to recognize your humanity, honour your journey, and nurture the care you so generously give.

Holding Space for Yourself: The Radical Act of Self-Compassion

You have mastered the art of creating sacred, non-judgmental spaces for your clients, patients, or loved ones. Now, imagine turning that same compassion inward.

Holding space for yourself means allowing all your feelings to be there—the joy, the pain, the exhaustion, and the hope—without rushing to fix or minimize them. It means giving yourself permission to be imperfect, to rest when you need it, and to ask for support without shame.

This is radical because so often, caregivers are conditioned to put others first, sometimes at the expense of their own wellbeing. But self-compassion is not selfish; it is foundational.

Try this: at the end of each day, pause and ask yourself, "What am I feeling right now? What do I need?" Listen without judgment. Hold whatever comes up with kindness, just as you would for a dear friend.

The Power and Necessity of Collective Care

Burnout and compassion fatigue don't thrive in isolation. They flourish when caregivers feel alone, unsupported, or unseen.

But healing is amplified when it happens in community.

Collective care means sharing your struggles and triumphs with others who understand the emotional landscape you walk. It means building networks of mutual support where vulnerabilities are met with empathy rather than judgment.

Whether it is a peer supervision group, a trusted circle of colleagues, or informal friendships, these connections are lifelines. They remind us that we are not alone, that our experiences are valid, and that healing is possible.

In communities, the weight of care is shared, and resilience is strengthened.

A Love Letter to the Weary Heart

Dear weary heart,

You have given so much. You have been the light in others' darkness, the steady hand in turbulent times. But what about your own light? What about your own peace?

Please remember, your worth is not tied to how much you give or how tirelessly you work. You are inherently worthy—simply because you are.

It is okay to say no. It is okay to slow down. It is okay to put yourself first sometimes.

Your compassion is a precious gift, but so is your healing.

Allow yourself to rest, to heal, to rediscover joy.

You deserve kindness—the same kindness you so freely offer.

With deep love and respect,

You.

Reflection Prompts to Hold Your Journey

- When was the last time you truly held space for your own feelings? What came up?

- Who in your life or work community helps you feel supported and seen? How can you deepen those connections?

- What are the messages of kindness you most need to hear from yourself right now?

- How might your healing enrich not only your life but also your ability to hold space for others?

- What boundaries can you set or refresh today that honour your limits and your care?

Practical Suggestions for Sustaining Yourself as a Caregiver

Create Ritual Pauses: Before and after your work—whether sessions with clients or caregiving moments—take intentional pauses. Breathe deeply, ground yourself, and release any emotional residue. These small rituals help you transition between your caregiving role and your personal self.

Set Compassionate Boundaries: Be clear about your availability and limits. Boundaries protect your energy and preserve your ability to give care sustainably. Remember, setting boundaries is an act of kindness to yourself and those you serve.

Engage in Peer Support: Regularly seek out colleagues or mentors who understand the emotional weight of your work. Peer supervision or informal check-ins provide a safe space to share burdens, gain perspective, and feel less isolated.

Prioritize Professional Self-Care: Therapy, coaching, or supervision for yourself is not optional—it is essential. These supports help you process your experiences and maintain mental and emotional health.

Celebrate Your Wins: Acknowledge and honour the small, daily acts of care and resilience. These victories remind you of your strength and dedication, even on challenging days.

Embracing Your Humanity: The Gift of Imperfection

Remember, being a healer doesn't require perfection. In fact, your authenticity—your willingness to be imperfect, vulnerable, and human—is what makes you truly powerful.

Clients and loved ones often find comfort not just in your knowledge or skills, but in your genuine presence. Your own journey through pain and healing can inspire hope and courage in others.

So be gentle with yourself when you falter. Know that every step you take—no matter how small—is meaningful.

Looking Ahead with Hope and Compassion

The path of caregiving and healing Is both challenging and profoundly rewarding. It asks a lot, but it also gives back in ways that enrich your soul.

As you continue this journey, may you hold yourself with the same kindness, patience, and compassion you offer to others.

Conclusion: Embracing the Quiet Strength Within

As we close this book, I want to honour the incredible journey you've been on—one filled with courage, honesty, and a deep desire to heal.

Burnout and compassion fatigue are not signs of weakness or failure. They are signals from your body, mind, and spirit telling you that something needs to change. Listening to these signals is the first step toward reclaiming your wellbeing.

Recovery is not a straight path. It is a winding, sometimes messy process with ups, downs, pauses, and leaps forward. And that's okay. What matters is that you keep moving gently toward healing, at your own pace, with kindness toward yourself.

You have already shown remarkable strength simply by acknowledging your struggles and seeking understanding. That quiet unravelling you've experienced holds the seeds of transformation—a chance to rebuild your life and work in ways that nourish and sustain you.

Remember, you are not alone in this. There is a community of hearts and hands holding you, rooting for your recovery and growth.

May you find rest without guilt, boundaries without fear, and joy in the everyday moments.

May you reclaim your story and rediscover the radiant, compassionate human at your core.

Above all, may you walk forward with gentle strength, knowing that healing is possible, and that you are deeply worthy of it.

Thank you for trusting yourself to embark on this path. The world is better because of your care—and because you are choosing to care for yourself, too.

With all my heart,
Andrea

Author's Note

Writing *The Quiet Unravelling* has been a deeply personal and meaningful journey for me. Like many of you, I have walked the winding road of burnout and compassion fatigue—not as a perfect expert, but as someone learning to understand, heal, and grow.

This book is born from my own experiences, from the stories shared by countless therapists, nurses, and caregivers I have had the honour to meet, and from the evolving research that shines a light on this misunderstood struggle.

To every reader holding this book, thank you for your courage to look honestly at your own experience. Thank you for choosing to give yourself the gift of care and kindness.

I am profoundly grateful to the many mentors, colleagues, friends, and loved ones who supported me along the way—your wisdom, encouragement, and compassion made this work possible.

A special thank you to Louise Daniels for allowing me to use the photo by Dylan Proctor of her sculpture Unravelling 2, which I'm sure you'll agree is the perfect cover for this book.

To the communities of caregivers around the world: keep holding space for one another. Together, we can change the conversation around burnout and build a culture that honours healing and human connection.

If you ever feel alone in this journey, please remember that your story matters—and help is always within reach.

With deepest gratitude and warmth,
Andrea Pluck

Further Reading & Resources

For those interested in exploring more about burnout, compassion fatigue, and self-care, here are some valuable resources:

Books:

Burnout: The Secret to Unlocking the Stress Cycle by Emily Nagoski and Amelia Nagoski

Compassion Fatigue: Coping with Secondary Traumatic Stress Disorder in Those Who Treat the Traumatized by Charles R. Figley

Radical Acceptance by Tara Brach

Articles & Journals:

Maslach, C., & Leiter, M. P. (2016). Understanding the burnout experience: Recent research and its implications. *Journal of Occupational Health Psychology*, 22(3), 254-262.

Figley, C. R. (2020). Compassion fatigue in health professionals: Introduction. *Journal of Trauma & Treatment*, 9(3), 1-7.

Online Resources:

The Compassion Fatigue Awareness Project (www.compassionfatigue.org)

Australian Psychological Society – Resources on burnout and self-care (www.psychology.org.au)

Mindful.org – Guided meditations and articles on mindfulness and self-compassion

Support Networks:

Peer supervision groups or professional associations in your field

Local or online caregiver support communities

Mental health professionals specialising in burnout and trauma recovery

Remember, seeking support and continuing education are vital steps on your healing journey.

References

American Psychiatric Association. (2022). Diagnostic and statistical manual of mental disorders (5th ed., text rev.). https://doi.org/10.1176/appi.books.9780890425787

Figley, C. R. (2002). Compassion fatigue: Psychotherapists' chronic lack of self-care. Brunner-Routledge.

Hersey, T. (2022). Rest is resistance: A manifesto. Little, Brown Spark.

Huggard, P., Stamm, B. H., & Pearlman, L. A. (2022). Compassion fatigue and burnout: Prevalence and prevention among caregivers. Clinical Psychology Review, 97, 102177. https://doi.org/10.1016/j.cpr.2022.102177

Maslach, C., & Leiter, M. P. (2016). Burnout: A multidimensional perspective. In R. J. Burke & C. L. Cooper (Eds.), The Routledge companion to wellbeing at work (pp. 47–59). Routledge.

Sinclair, S., Raffin-Bouchal, S., Venturato, L., et al. (2017). Compassion fatigue: A meta-narrative review of the healthcare literature. International Journal of

Nursing Studies, 69, 9–24. https://doi.org/10.1016/j.ijnurstu.2017.01.003

West, C. P., Dyrbye, L. N., Erwin, P. J., & Shanafelt, T. D. (2018). Interventions to prevent and reduce physician burnout: A systematic review and meta-analysis. The Lancet, 388(10057), 2272–2281. https://doi.org/10.1016/S0140-6736(16)31279-X

World Health Organization. (2019). Burn-out an "occupational phenomenon": International Classification of Diseases. https://www.who.int/mental_health/evidence/burn-out/en/

Golkar, A., Johansson, E., Kasamatsu, T., Osika, W., Perski, A., & Savic, I. (2014). The influence of work-related chronic stress on the regulation of emotion and on functional connectivity in the brain. *PLOS ONE, 9*(9), e104550. https://doi.org/10.1371/journal.pone.0104550

Juster, R. P., McEwen, B. S., & Lupien, S. J. (2010). Allostatic load biomarkers of chronic stress and impact on health and cognition. *Neuroscience & Biobehavioral Reviews, 35*(1), 2–16. https://doi.org/10.1016/j.neubiorev.2009.10.002

Konturek, P. C., Brzozowski, T., & Konturek, S. J. (2011). Stress and the gut: Pathophysiology, clinical consequences, diagnostic approach and treatment options. *Journal of Physiology and Pharmacology*, *62*(6), 591–599.

McEwen, B. S. (2004). Protection and damage from acute and chronic stress: Allostasis and allostatic overload and relevance to the pathophysiology of psychiatric disorders. *Annals of the New York Academy of Sciences*, *1032*, 1–7. https://doi.org/10.1196/annals.1314.001

Meerlo, P., Sgoifo, A., & Suchecki, D. (2008). Restricted and disrupted sleep: Effects on autonomic function, neuroendocrine stress systems and stress responsivity. *Sleep Medicine Reviews*, *12*(3), 197–210. https://doi.org/10.1016/j.smrv.2007.07.007

Porges, S. W. (2011). *The polyvagal theory: Neurophysiological foundations of emotions, attachment, communication, and self-regulation*. Norton.

Savic, I. (2015). Structural changes of the brain in relation to occupational stress. *Cerebral Cortex*, *25*(6), 1554–1564. https://doi.org/10.1093/cercor/bht348

Streeter, C. C., Gerbarg, P. L., Saper, R. B., Ciraulo, D. A., & Brown, R. P. (2012). Effects of yoga on the autonomic nervous system, gamma-aminobutyric-acid, and allostasis in epilepsy, depression, and post-traumatic stress disorder. *Medical Hypotheses, 78*(5), 571–579. https://doi.org/10.1016/j.mehy.2012.01.021

Hochschild, A. R. (1983). *The managed heart: Commercialization of human feeling.* University of California Press.

Singer, T., & Klimecki, O. M. (2014). Empathy and compassion. *Current Biology, 24*(18), R875–R878. https://doi.org/10.1016/j.cub.2014.06.054

Mealer, M., Burnham, E. L., Coode, C. J., Rothbaum, B., & Moss, M. (2009). The prevalence and impact of post-traumatic stress disorder and burnout syndrome in nurses. *Depression and Anxiety, 26*(12), 1118-1126. https://doi.org/10.1002/da.20631

Sorenson, C., Bolick, B., Wright, K., & Hamilton, R. (2016). Understanding compassion fatigue in healthcare providers: A review of current literature. *Journal of Nursing Scholarship, 48*(5), 456-465. https://doi.org/10.1111/jnu.12229

Shanafelt, T. D., & Noseworthy, J. H. (2017). Executive leadership and physician well-being: Nine organizational strategies to promote engagement and reduce burnout. Mayo Clinic Proceedings, 92(1), 129-146. https://doi.org/10.1016/j.mayocp.2016.10.004

West, C. P., Dyrbye, L. N., & Shanafelt, T. D. (2018). Physician burnout: contributors, consequences and solutions. Journal of Internal Medicine, 283(6), 516-529. https://doi.org/10.1111/joim.12752

Lee, H., & Miller, L. (2022). Boundaries and burnout: The importance of self-care in caregiving professions. *Journal of Occupational Health Psychology, 27*(4), 341-355. https://doi.org/10.1037/ocp0000312

Rupert, P. A., & Morgan, D. J. (2005). Work setting and burnout among professional psychologists. *Professional Psychology: Research and Practice, 36*(5), 544-550. https://doi.org/10.1037/0735-7028.36.5.544

Baker, F. C., & Driver, H. S. (2013). Circadian rhythms, sleep, and the timing of physiological events. *Sleep Medicine Clinics,* 8(4), 417–431. https://doi.org/10.1016/j.jsmc.2013.06.005

Cacioppo, J. T., & Patrick, W. (2008). *Loneliness: Human nature and the need for social connection.* W. W. Norton & Company.

Field, T. (2016). Yoga research review. *Complementary Therapies in Clinical Practice*, 24, 145-161. https://doi.org/10.1016/j.ctcp.2016.06.005

Kabat-Zinn, J. (2005). *Wherever you go, there you are: Mindfulness meditation in everyday life*. Hachette Books.

Lehrer, P., Eddie, D., & Sloan, R. P. (2020). Biofeedback and heart rate variability: A primer for clinical practice. *Applied Psychophysiology and Biofeedback*, 45, 145-162. https://doi.org/10.1007/s10484-019-09446-9

Roenneberg, T. (2019). *Internal time: Chronotypes, social jet lag, and why you are so tired*. Harvard University Press.

Support in Australia

If you are feeling overwhelmed, emotionally exhausted, or just need someone to talk to, please know that support is available—and you are absolutely worthy of it.

Whether you are struggling with burnout, compassion fatigue, anxiety, or low mood, the following services offer confidential, professional help:

Beyond Blue
Support for anxiety, depression, and emotional wellbeing
1300 22 4636 (24/7)
www.beyondblue.org.au

Lifeline Australia
Crisis support and suicide prevention
13 11 14 (24/7)
www.lifeline.org.au

QLife
Support for LGBTQIA+ people
1800 184 527 (3 pm – midnight daily)
www.qlife.org.au

Nurse & Midwife Support

Free, confidential support for nurses, midwives, and students

1800 667 877 (24/7)

www.nmsupport.org.au

Mental Health Professionals Network

Connects health professionals to peer support and mental health resources

www.mhpn.org.au

Your GP

Don't forget: your general practitioner can be a vital part of your support team. They can help you create a mental health care plan and refer you to psychologists, counsellors, or other specialists.

You don't have to navigate this alone. Please reach out if you are struggling. Help is here—and so is hope.

For International Readers

Wherever you are in the world, your mental health matters. If you are feeling overwhelmed, numb, anxious, or exhausted, please know this: support exists, and reaching out is an act of courage—not weakness.

Below are some global mental health services and directories that may help you find support in your area.

Befrienders Worldwide
Offers emotional support and suicide prevention through a network of helplines in over 30 countries
Find your local helpline: www.befrienders.org

International Association for Suicide Prevention (IASP)
Resources and crisis centre contacts around the world
www.iasp.info/resources/Crisis_Centres/

Samaritans (UK & Ireland)
Emotional support for anyone in distress
116 123 (24/7, free in UK and Ireland)
www.samaritans.org

National Suicide Prevention Lifeline (USA)
988 (24/7)
www.988lifeline.org

Talk Suicide Canada
1-833-456-4566 (24/7)
www.talksuicide.ca

Mental Health Foundation of New Zealand
www.mentalhealth.org.nz

Not sure where to turn?

If you are in crisis or feeling unsafe, you can also go to your nearest hospital emergency department or contact your local emergency services.

Please take care of yourself. Even in your most depleted moments, you are deserving of rest, of support, and of a life that feels like your own again.

Other publications by Andrea Pluck

If you found comfort and clarity in *The Quiet Unravelling*, you may also enjoy Andrea's other work, including:

Moments - A Collection of Tiny Thoughts

A beautifully crafted collection of reflections, affirmations, and quiet wisdom not only for those navigating the cancer experience—offering hope, calm, and comfort, one tiny thought at a time.

From Self-Doubt to Confidence - Understanding Imposter Syndrome

Written especially for helping professionals, this book untangles the knot of not-enoughness. It offers insight, relatable stories, and actionable strategies to quiet the inner critic and reconnect with your professional worth.

Andrea also teaches several popular online courses grounded in compassion and real-world relevance.

Each book and course are a small offering of care from someone who's walked the path and continues to learn, stumble, and grow—just like you.